A Checkup with the Doctor

by Katherine A. Smith

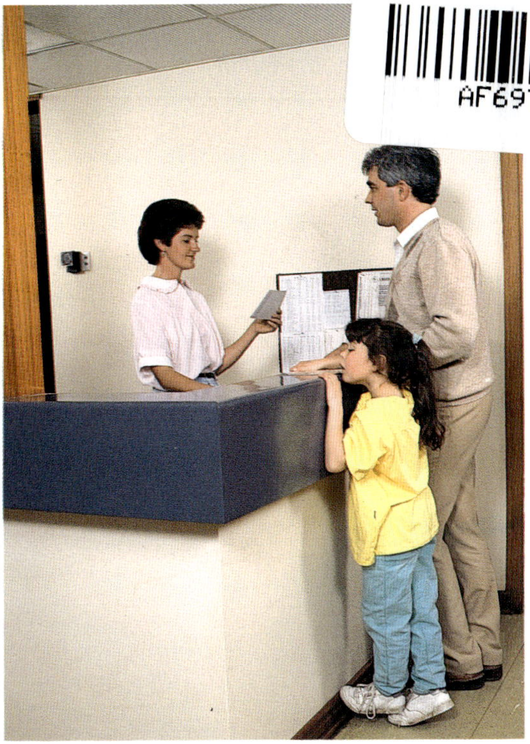

McDougal, Littell & Company
Evanston, Illinois
New York Dallas Sacramento Raleigh

MAGIC BEAN IN-FACT SERIES

Contents

About This Book

This book shows what happens when you go for a checkup. These are some of the instruments the doctor might use to examine you.

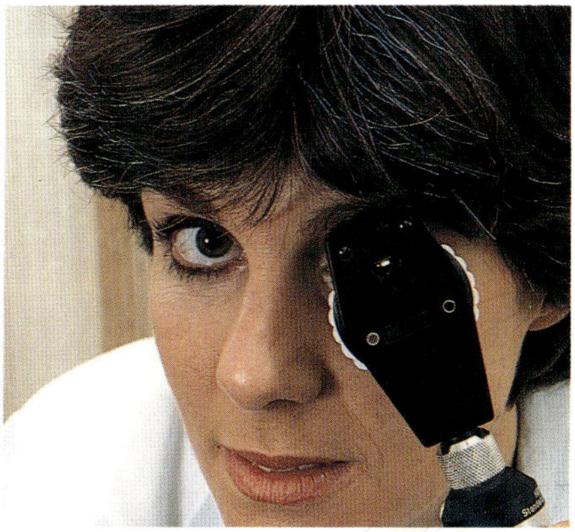

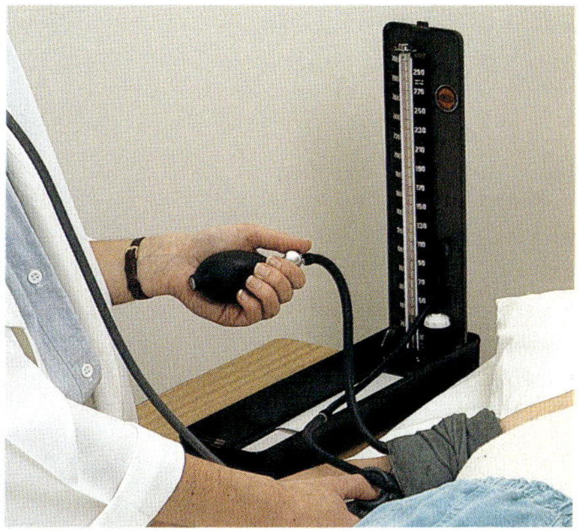

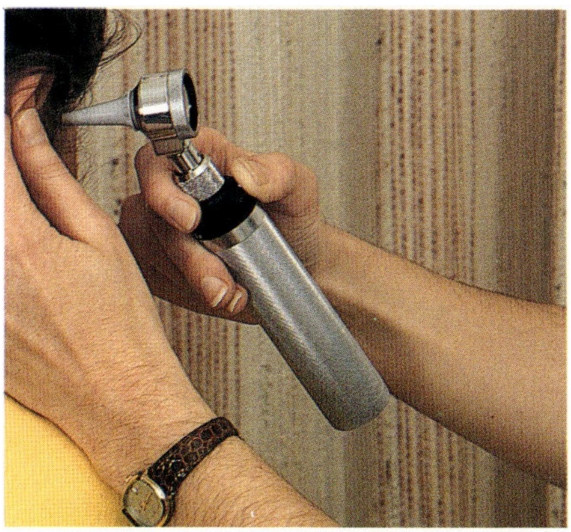

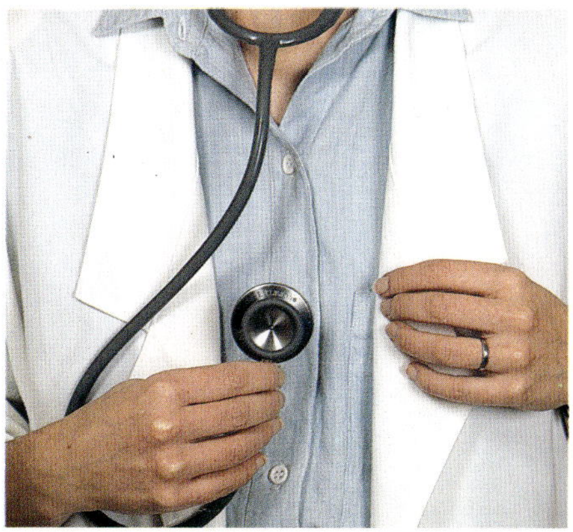

Measuring Stick and Scale

The doctor uses a measuring stick to see how tall you are. She records your height and checks how much you have grown.

The doctor asks you to stand on the scale to record your weight. She will use this information to monitor your growth rate.

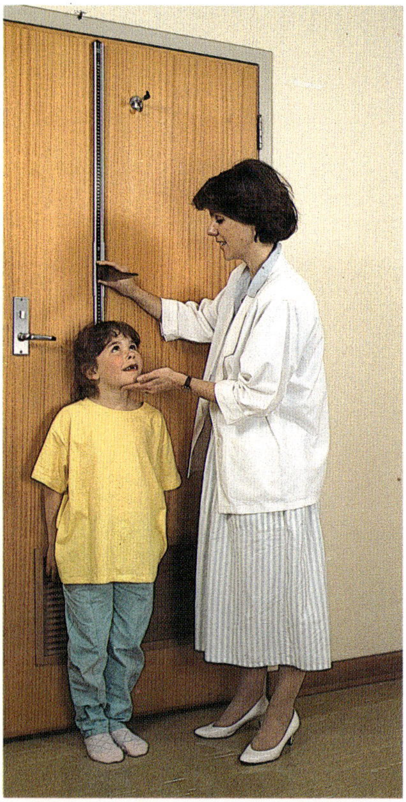

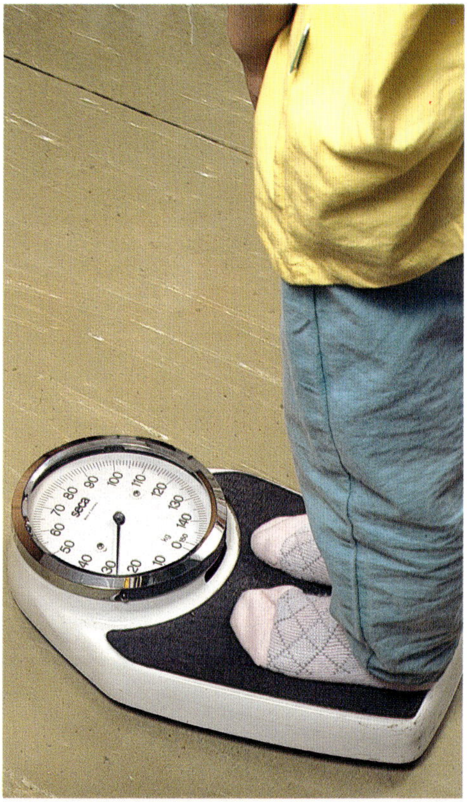

Tongue Depressor

A tongue depressor looks like a large ice-cream stick. The doctor puts it on top of your tongue and asks you to say *Ah.* When you say *Ah*, your tongue automatically moves out of the way so that she can see the pharynx, tonsils, and palate. With a light the doctor checks whether your tonsils are swollen or inflamed.

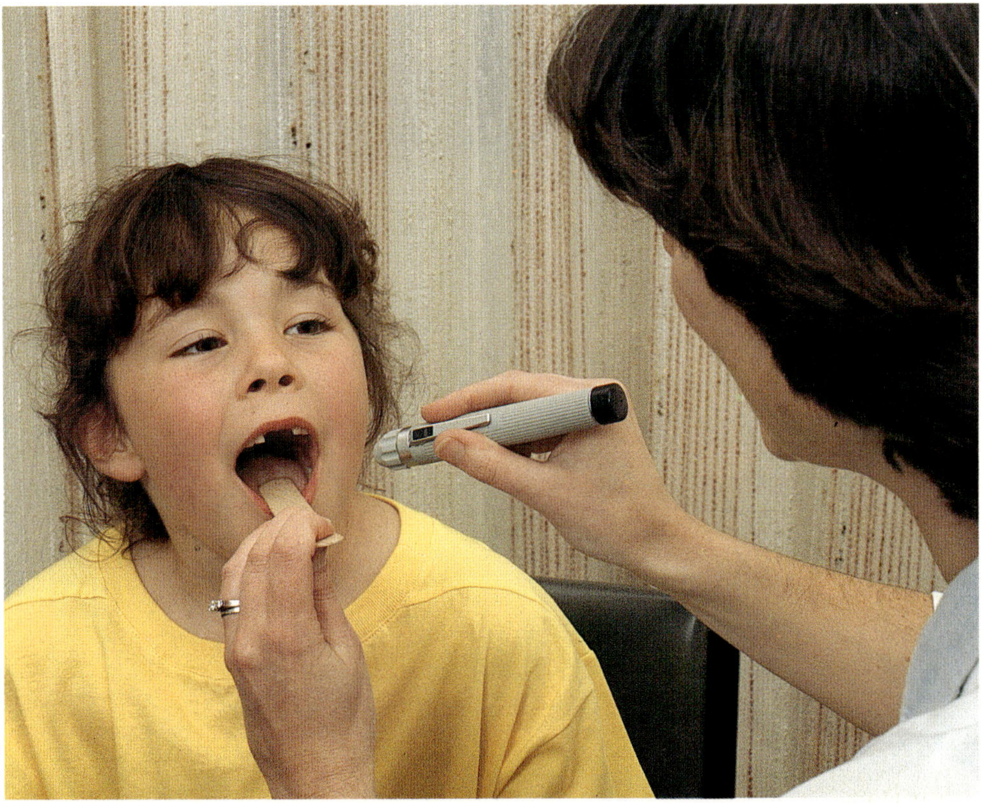

Oroscope (**or**ra-skope)

The doctor uses an oroscope to look inside your ears. (See diagram, opposite page.) It has a little light on the end and a lens, which makes the eardrum look several times larger. If the eardrum is red or swollen, you may have an infection.

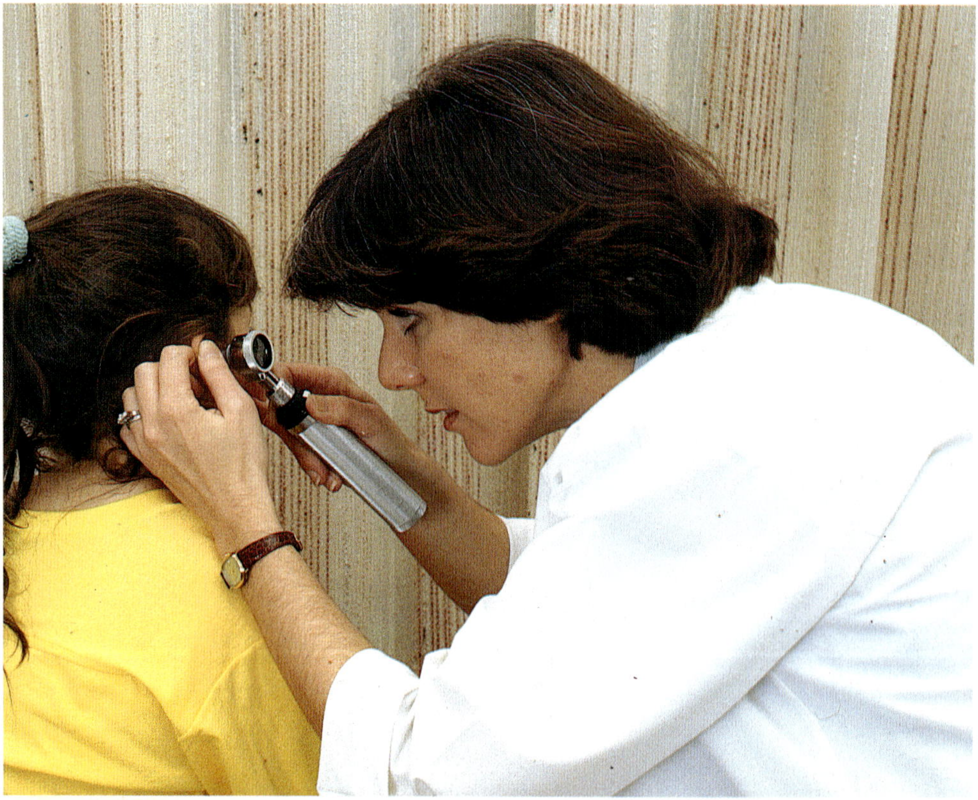

Inside the Ear

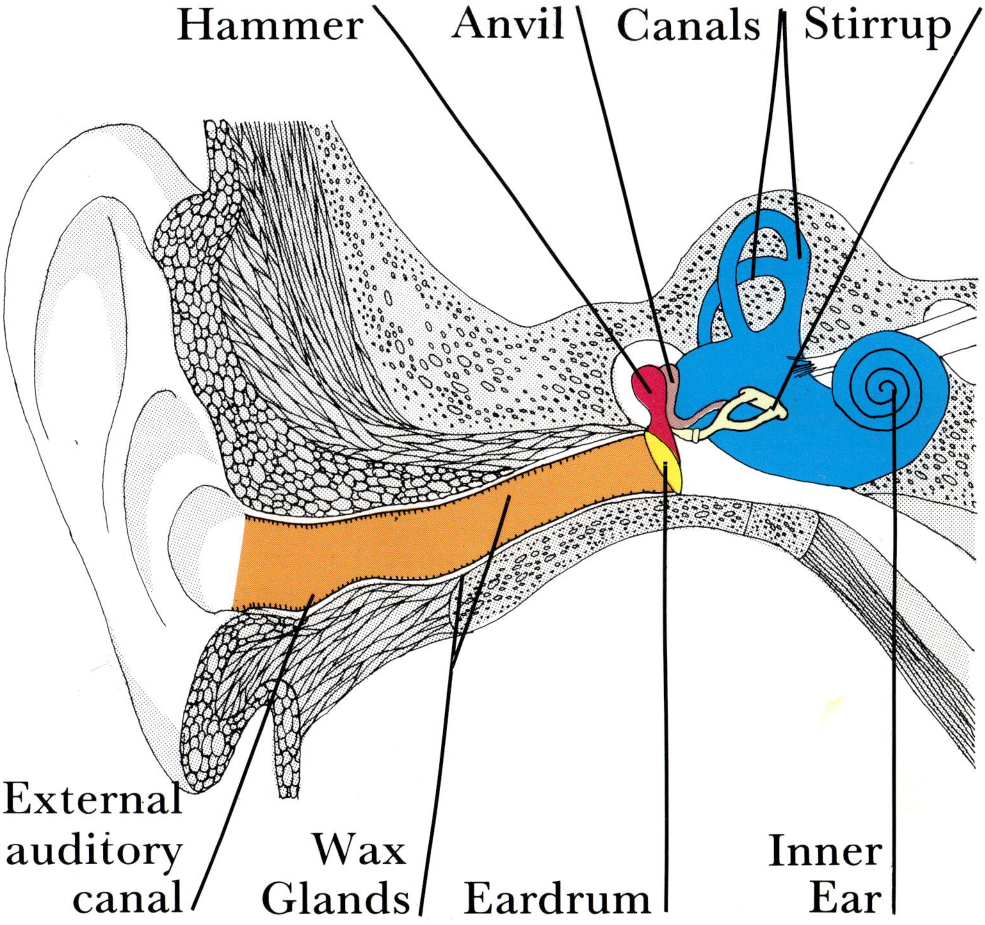

Ophthalmoscope (off-**thal**mo-skope)

The doctor uses an ophthalmoscope to look inside your eyes. (See diagram, opposite page.) She can see the back of your eye with the magnifying lens. The doctor also checks the movement of your pupils by shining a light onto them and watching to see if they become smaller.

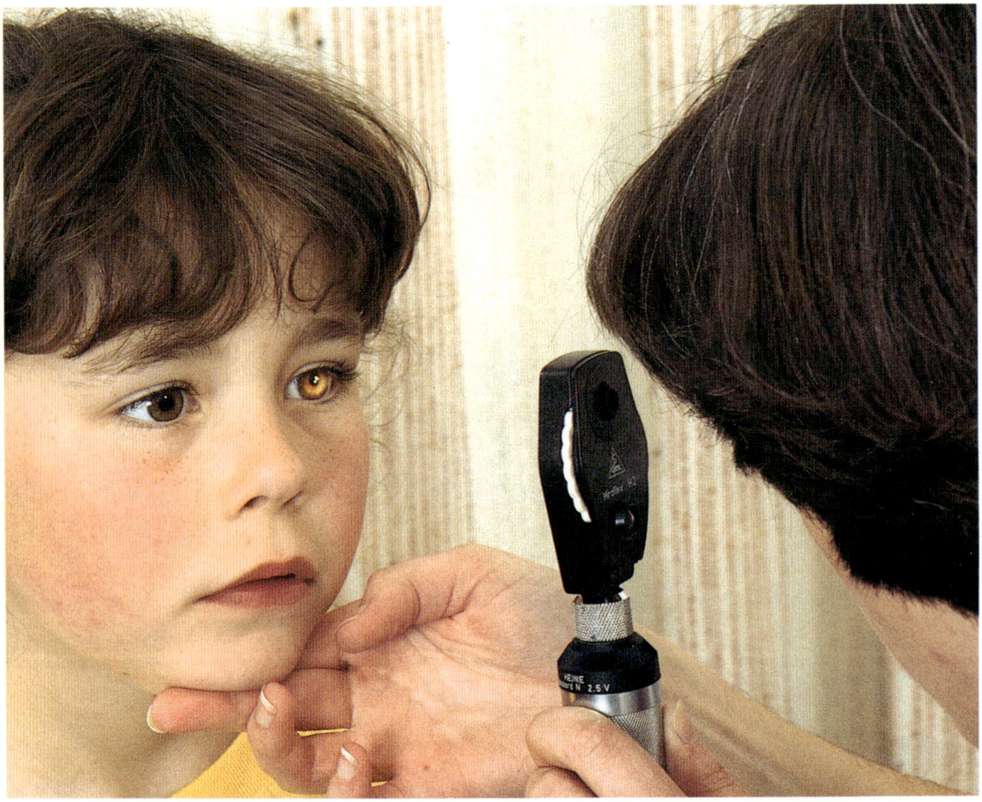

Inside the Eye

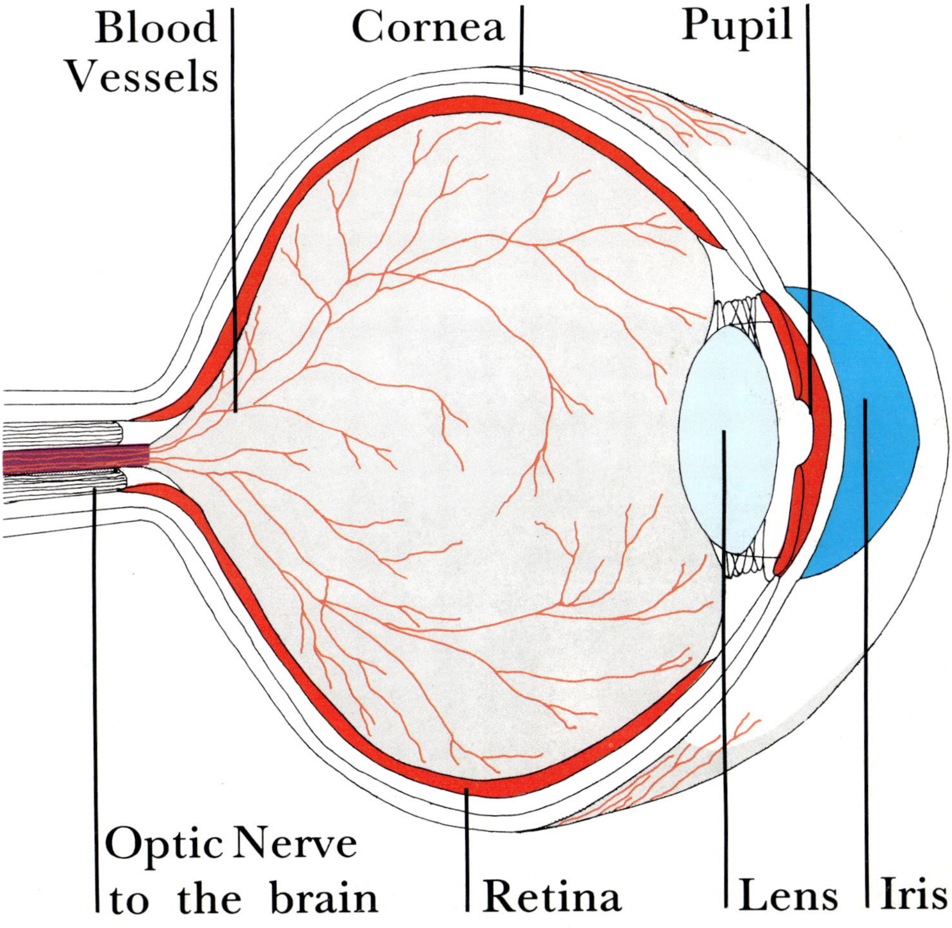

Eye Chart

The doctor uses an eye chart to check how sharp your vision is. You have to read each line from left to right. The symbols start off large but get smaller and smaller as you read down the chart. The symbols on the chart can be shapes or letters.

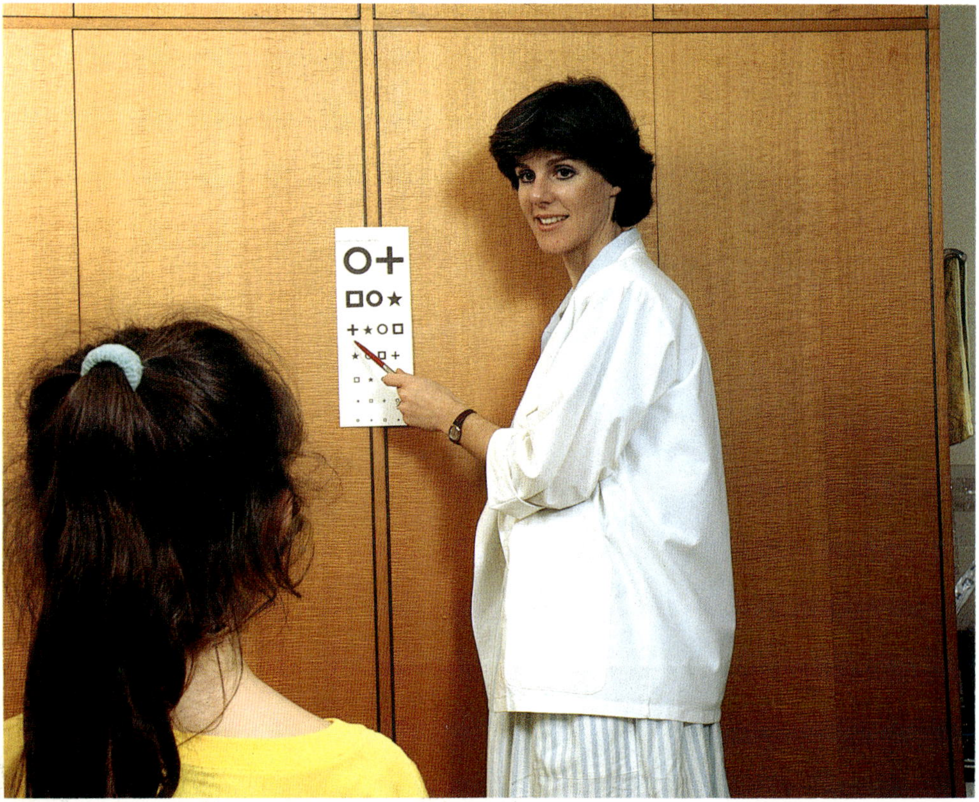

Thermometer (ther-**mom**mi-ter)

A thermometer is a thin tube the doctor uses to take your temperature. A normal temperature is 98.6°F (37.2° C). She puts the thermometer in your mouth or under your arm for at least two minutes. If your temperature is 99°F (37.5°C) or higher you may have an infection.

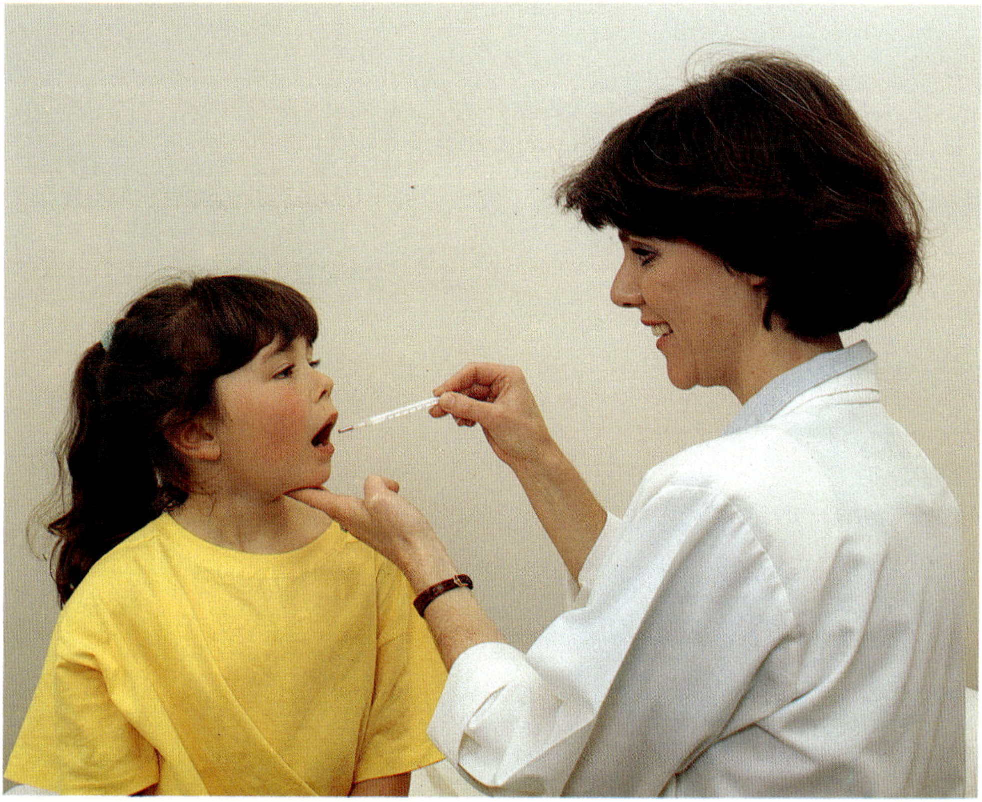

Stethoscope (**steth**a-skope)

The doctor uses a stethoscope to check your heartbeat and your breathing. She places it over your lungs to listen for normal breathing sounds. The doctor also puts the stethoscope over your heart to check that it is making the regular *boom-boom, boom-boom* sound.

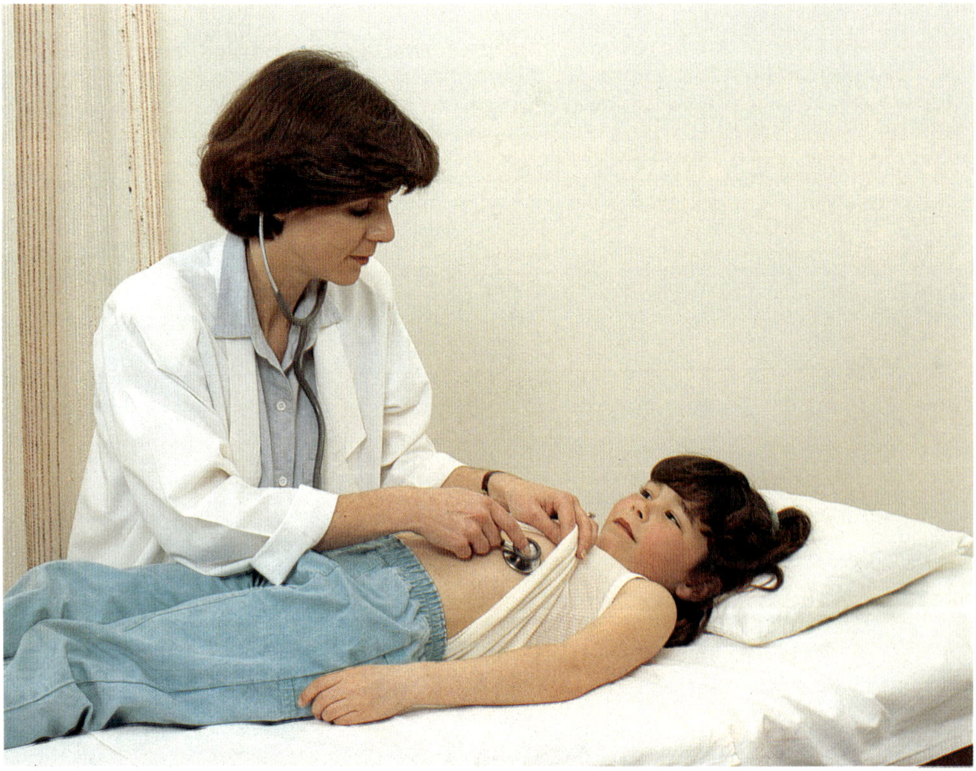

Sphygmomanometer

(**sfig**mo-man-**om**mi-ter)

The doctor uses a sphygmomanometer to check your blood pressure. She wraps a firm bandage around your arm. Then she pumps air into the bandage and it gets tighter. The doctor reads the pressure gauge and listens for the *boom-boom* of blood being pumped by the heart.

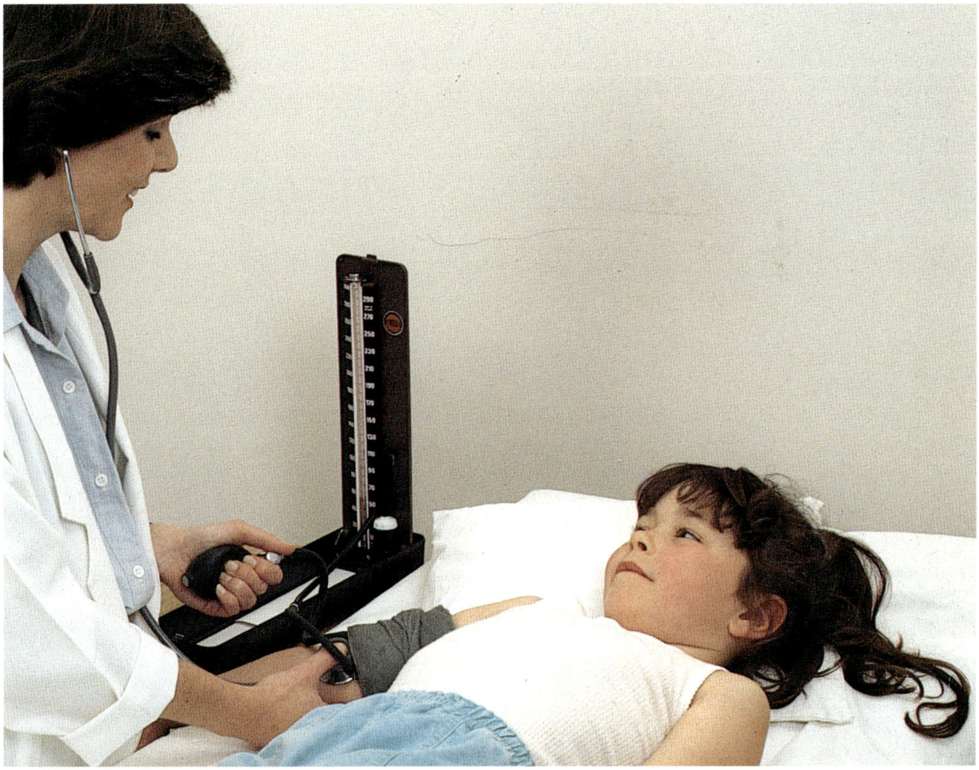

Reflex Hammer

The doctor uses a reflex hammer to see if your tendons, muscles, and nerves are working properly. She uses it on the tendons of joints such as the ankle, knee, elbow, and wrist. As the doctor hits a tendon with the hammer, the muscles quickly shorten. This makes your limb jump.

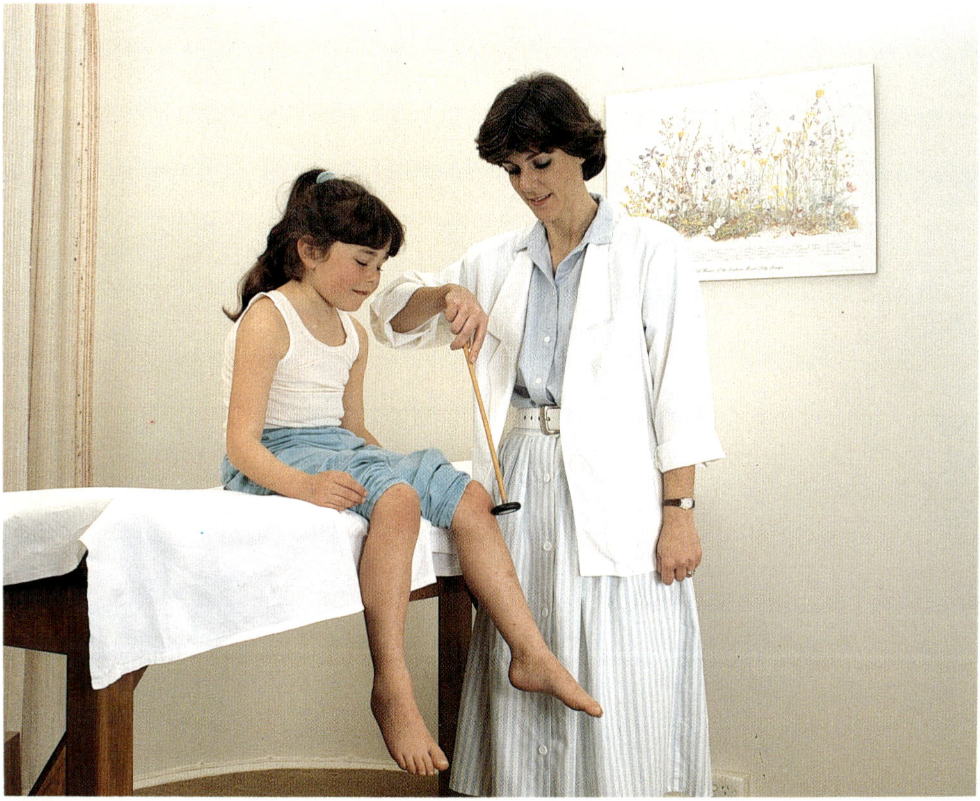

Injection

The doctor gives a shot, or injection, to cure or protect you from illness. An injection that protects you is called *immunization* and prevents diseases such as measles, mumps, diphtheria and tetanus. She uses a syringe and needle. The syringe has the medicine in it.

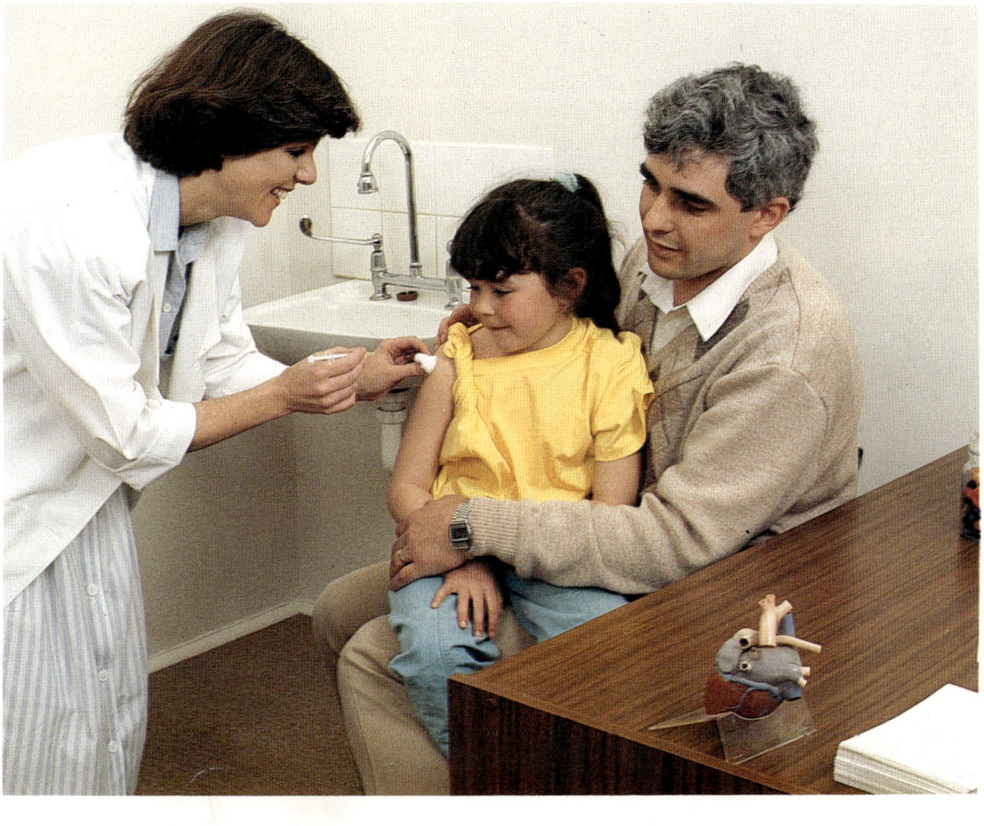

Record Card

When a checkup is over the doctor notes symptoms, problems, and treatments on your special record card.

KINGSWAY CLINIC

Hampton Susie 1/13/83
31 Greentree Rd Belair
2/2/87 4½ Fall from swing laceration 3inches forehead
Xylocoline 2% 3NC Clean with Betadine
Sutured 12x4/0 prolene ROS 1/52
1/19/88 5yo Vax CDT & POLIO
4/22/88 5 3/12 Mo concerned re vision
O/E Acuity 6/6 (L)
6/12 (R)
Squint noted Rx Ref Ophthalmologist
7/12/88 5 5/12 Tonsillitis & Nodes & Fever R Amoxil
1/15/89 6yo Checkup.

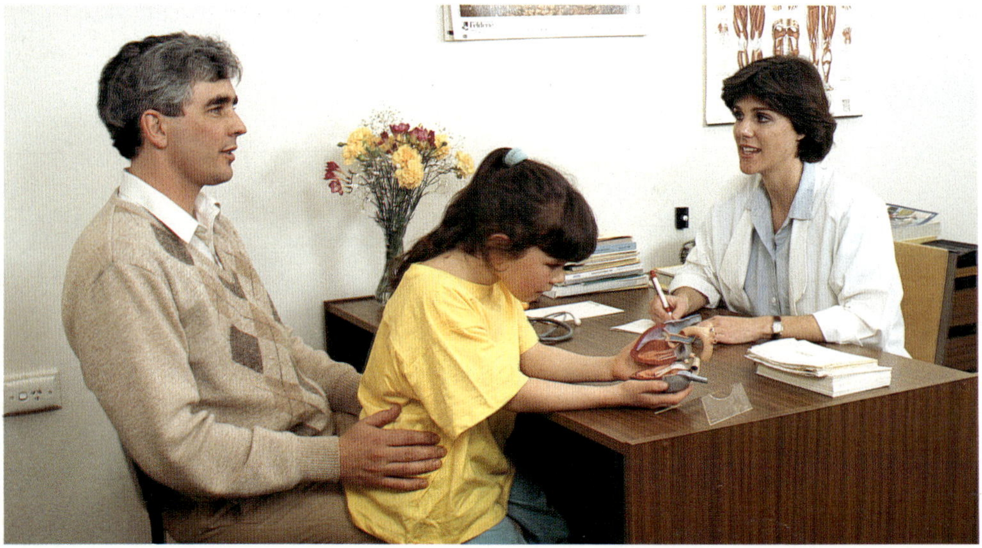